The Complete Raw Food Diet Guide

Lose Weight Quickly, Achieve Optimal Health and Feel Energized with the Raw Food Diet and Raw Food Recipes

EMMA ROSE

Table of Contents

Introduction

I want to thank you and congratulate you for purchasing this book!

This book contains proven steps and strategies on how to effectively apply the raw food diet into your life.

A raw food diet, also known as uncooked diet, is essentially an eating plan that largely involves the consumption of unprocessed and uncooked food. Those who take on this lifestyle are often acknowledged as raw foodists or raw food practitioners. Sometimes, they are referred to as raw food advocates, although this term may also be used to individuals who are interested in or about to convert to the raw food diet.

In the diet, it is believed that cooking or heating of food will destroy the natural enzymes and nutrients typically found in food and produce. This can bring about complications because these enzymes are mainly responsible for fighting off diseases and improving digestion. Therefore, in order to avoid this, raw foodists eat food in its raw state, as the diet's name suggests. This helps alkalize the body, since cooked food has acidic toxins that disrupt the body's acid/alkaline balance. Such disruption often causes illnesses and excess weight. In a nutshell, heating food above 118°F initiates the chemical changes that produce the acidic toxins like free radicals, mutagens and carcinogens, which are normally linked to diseases such as heart problems, arthritis, cancer and diabetes.

There are more than one variations of the diet, and it is entirely up to you how you will shape up your own diet plan. Generally, to be considered a raw foodist, an individual must at least eat 75% to 100% raw, unprocessed and organic food and drink pure water. Most of the items you will eat are plant-based which should never be heated above 115°F. While majority of raw foodists are vegetarian, there are those who opt to consume raw animal products such as raw fish, sashimi, raw milk and the like. Some may also incorporate fresh fruits and vegetables into their meal plan. On the whole, you have the power to create whatever raw food diet structure suits your lifestyle and your preferences best.

Thanks again for purchasing this book, I hope you enjoy it! Please take some time to stop by and LIKE our Facebook page:

https://www.facebook.com/joypublishing

With gratitude,

Emma Rose

Chapter 1

An Overview of the Raw Food Diet

The concept of the raw food diet is simple – cooking diminishes the nutritional value of food. Even though most of the food items in the diet are consumed while it is raw, heating is acceptable provided that the temperature stays between the range of 104 to 118°F or below.

Since cooking is perceived to kill off enzymes naturally found in food, raw food practitioners choose to avoid cooked food. As a matter of fact, overconsumption of cooked food forces the body to work overtime in order to produce more enzymes to support normal bodily functions. In the long run, the lack of enzymes can instigate a lot of problems involving a person's health, particularly accelerated aging, nutrient deficiency, weight gain and digestive problems.

Going raw can prove to be challenging, especially for those that are just starting out. It takes a lot of discipline to stick to the principles of the diet. Moreover, extra effort is required mentally and physically. When it comes to preparing your daily raw meals, your options are limited. Here are some of the procedures you may apply when organizing your meal plan:

- *Germination* – this is the process of soaking in water for a certain period of time. The recommended amount of time differs from one person to another but for raw foodists, the safest bet is to soak overnight.

- *Sprouting* – this comes after germination. After the beans, legumes or seeds are soaked, they may then be sprouted. Items should be left at room temperature until a sprout comes out of it. These sprouts may then be used for preparing food but should be rinsed and drained thoroughly beforehand.

- *Blending* – involves the use of a blender or food processor in order to create sauces, smoothies, or soup among others.

- *Dehydrating* – employs an equipment known as a dehydrator, which simulates sun drying. Common products of dehydrators are crackers, croutons, raisins, fruit leathers, sundried tomatoes, breads and kale chips.

- *Pickling* – a method of preserving food by marinating in a brine.

- *Juicing* – the process of extracting of vitamins, minerals and natural juices from plant tissues, particularly raw fruits and vegetables.

- *Fermentation* – process of converting sugar to carbon dioxide through the use of yeast.

Now that you know what procedures are available to you when preparing your raw meals, the next thing to know is which particular equipment/s you need to use. Below are some of the staple equipment that can be seen in every raw foodist's kitchen:

- *Dehydrator* – it is an enclosed container that has heating elements that can warm at low temperatures. It has a fan that blows warm air onto the food.

- *Spiral Slicer* – slices vegetables into spiral shapes

- *Thermometer* – to ensure that temperature stays below 118°F when heating food.

- *Trays* – for soaking and sprouting beans, legumes or seeds

- *Sprouters* or *mason jars*

- *Food processor*

- *Blender*

- *Juicer*

These are the basic things you have to know if you intend to convert to the raw food diet. Now that you have an idea of what it is and how it works, you will then have to figure out why you would want to choose this lifestyle.

Chapter 2

Why Do People Go Raw?

To some people, converting to a raw food diet seems like a crazy idea. After all, why would anyone want to give up eating all the delectable cooked dishes for uncooked food? How could one survive solely on salads? Why should you limit your choices when eating? These are just some of the many questions people ask when it comes to changing up their diet. Truth be told, there is a less-than-enthusiastic reception from others. Despite these doubts and uncertainties about the diet, those who choose to go raw are very passionate about adhering to the lifestyle. In fact, raw food diet practitioners more often than not retain this routine for years or even for the rest of their lives.

For those who are wondering why someone would stick to such a challenging and demanding way of life, there are several reasons why people take on the diet. For most, optimal health is the primary objective. Some choose to uphold their philosophical and ethical principles. Then there are others who are merely drawn to the diet's environment-friendly quality. These objectives are further explained below.

Health Reasons

Perhaps the most typical reason why anyone would want to begin a raw food diet is the fact that it is beneficial to one's health. For one, it helps prevent and fight off diseases because of the abundance of vitamins, minerals, nutrients and antioxidants that help reduce risks of illnesses or slow down its progress. It also helps that raw food has a lack of calories, saturated fat, cholesterol and other possibly harmful elements normally found in cooked, processed food. Weight loss is also a huge motivation for raw foodists, since a raw diet rich in fiber and low in calories is a great, fast way to shed pounds. Overall, one's health and well-being is positively affected by the raw food diet.

Philosophical and Ethical Reasons

There are a number of individuals who prefer to apply raw food diet because it is in line with their philosophical and ethical beliefs and principles. These are the same people who refuse to purchase animal meat and processed food. As an alternative, these people choose to support organic agriculture and food coming from plants. A moral code like this is surprisingly a strong incentive for some to go raw.

Environmental Reasons

Environmental benefits were once viewed merely as a bonus as opposed to a primary purpose for going raw, particularly for raw vegan foodists. The cooking and processing of food items also have great effect on the environment. Gigantic amounts of resources are used in the food processing industry. Furthermore, most raw foodists encourage organic agriculture, hence using their money to buy food and advocate against the use of chemical fertilizers, herbicides and pesticides that can damage and eventually destroy the environment.

These are the principal reasons why an individual would want to apply the raw food diet and make it a part of his or her daily routine. Raw foodists have their own opinions and motives for considering such a lifestyle choice.

Chapter 3

Raw Food Recipes to Get You Started

This wide array of recipes will help you sustain a raw food diet without getting tired of eating the same food over and over again.

Sauces, Dressings and Condiments

Most meals are dull and boring without sauces and condiments. A delicious sauce can add more taste and flavor to a dish. However, some worry that by following a diet, one must ultimately give up the use of sauces and condiments. While you cannot use the traditional processed sauces, you may create your own using the recipes below.

1. Silica-Rich Dressing

Cucumbers are packed with the minerals responsible for nourishing connective tissues such as the nails, hair, bones and skin. Moreover, they are naturally refreshing and hydrating. By using cucumbers in this recipe, they allow oil reduction, which makes this dressing a low-calorie option.

Ingredients:

- 1 ¼ cups of cucumber, chopped, peeled and seeded
- 2 tablespoons of apple cider vinegar
- 1 tablespoon of flat-leaf parsley, chopped
- 1 small clove of garlic
- 2 teaspoons of cilantro, chopped
- ¼ cup of extra virgin olive oil
- ¼ teaspoon of dried dill
- ¼ teaspoon of ground black pepper
- ¼ teaspoon of ground red pepper
- ¼ teaspoon of salt

Procedure:

1. Add the cucumber, parsley, cilantro, garlic, vinegar, red pepper, black pepper, dill and salt to a blender or food processor. Blend until smooth.

2. While processing, slowly add the olive oil. Blend for at least 15 seconds or until the oil is fully absorbed.

3. Pour into a container and store in the refrigerator. Shake well before use.

2. Zucchini Hummus

This is similar to the traditional Middle Eastern version but with a highlight on zucchini, which is low on calories. It can be used as a dip, dressing or spread.

Ingredients:

- 1 ½ zucchinis, chopped
- 3 cloves of garlic
- ¾ cup of sesame seeds
- 1/3 cup of parsley, chopped
- 3 ½ tablespoons of lemon juice
- 1/3 teaspoon of salt

Procedure:

1. Blend seeds in a food processor until it achieves a peanut butter-like consistency (tahini). Set aside.

2. Mince the garlic using the food processor.

3. Add the zucchinis, salt, lemon juice and parsley. Process until crudely chopped.

4. Add the tahini to the processor. Blend until smooth.

3. Italian Herb Tomato Sauce

This sauce is easy to prepare and is much healthier. Tomatoes are also rich in several nutrients such as vitamins A and C, folic acid and lycopene. By making the sauce naturally, you get to take advantage of the nutrients that the tomatoes supply. This sauce will go well with other recipes.

Ingredients:

- 2 ½ cups of fresh tomatoes, chopped
- ¼ cup of sun-dried tomatoes
- 2 ½ teaspoon of dried Italian herbs (e.g. oregano, basil, rosemary and parsley)
- 1 clove of garlic
- ½ celery stalk
- 1/3 teaspoon of salt

Procedure:

1. Soak the sun-dried tomatoes preferably overnight or at for at least 2 hours in water until soft.

2. Mince the herbs, salt, garlic and celery in a food processor.

3. Add the soaked sun-dried tomatoes. Blend well and set aside in a large bowl.

4. Place the chopped fresh tomatoes in food processor and process until chunky and saucy.

5. Add to the sun-dried tomato paste. Stir and mix until fully combined.

4. Soured Coconut Cream

Sour cream is a classic dip found in American and European cuisine. This version utilizes coconut to ensure you stick to your diet. It has a tangy taste plus all the healthy nutrients found in coconuts.

Ingredients:

- ¾ cup of fresh young coconut meat
- 2 teaspoons of lemon juice
- ½ teaspoon of onion powder
- ½ teaspoon of garlic powder
- ½ cup of water

Procedure:

1. Using a blender or food processor, blend all the ingredients until smooth and faintly whipped.

2. Place finished product in a lidded glass jar. Refrigerate.

5. Rawbecue Sauce

This is the raw version of the barbecue sauce and can work well either as a marinade, dip or dressing.

Ingredients:

- 1 dried pepper, soaked
- 1 clove of garlic
- 1 cup of sundried tomatoes, soaked
- 1 cup of fresh tomato, chopped
- 2 tablespoons of yacon syrup
- 2 tablespoons of apple cider vinegar
- 2 teaspoons of chili powder
- 1 teaspoon of nama shoyu
- ½ teaspoon of salt
- ½ cup of soaking water

Procedure:

1. In a blender, place all the ingredients together. Blend until smooth.

2. Store the finished sauce in a glass jar with a lid. Refrigerate.

Breakfast

Considered the most important meal of the day, breakfast is the perfect time for raw food enthusiasts to enjoy meals, from fruits and vegetables to classic breakfast meals with a raw twist. A nutritious meal will allow you to retain your energy throughout the day.

1. Walnut Banana Pancakes

Pancakes are a breakfast favorite, and this recipe allows you to enjoy this childhood favorite and still staying true to the raw food diet. Sadly, this is not the kind of pancake that you can make instantly just by mixing.

Ingredients:

- 6 bananas, sliced
- 2 apples, chopped and cored
- 1 ½ cups of buckwheat
- 1 tablespoon of flax seeds
- 1 cup of sunflower seeds
- 2 tablespoons of coconut flakes
- ½ cup of walnuts, chopped
- 1 ¼ tablespoons of ground cinnamon
- ¼ teaspoon of salt

Procedure:

1. Soak the sunflower seeds and buckwheat overnight or for no less than 6 hours. Rinse well before use.

2. In a coffee grinder or blender, process the flax seeds until it turns into powder. Set aside.

3. In a food processor, blend sunflower seeds and buckwheat until it gets a creamy consistency. Place in a bowl.

4. Process the bananas, apples, salt and cinnamon until smooth. Add to the bowl.

5. Add the walnuts, coconut flakes and flax seeds to the mixture. Mix thoroughly.

6. Prepare ParaFlexx sheets. Shape pancakes by hand. If you have a dehydrator, dehydrate the mixtures for 8 to 12 hours. Otherwise, use an oven until the mixture is dry on the outside but moist inside.

2. Breakfast Tacos with Ruby Raspberry Filling

The romaine lettuce contains antioxidants in its leaves that is said to help battle cancer. It also helps give this recipe a crunchy feel, which is exactly how tacos should be.

Ingredients:

- Breakfast Tacos with Ruby Raspberry Filling
- The romaine lettuce contains antioxidants in its leaves that is said to help battle cancer. It also helps give this recipe a crunchy feel, which is exactly how tacos should be.
- *Ingredients:*
- 4 to 8 romaine leaves
- 1 ruby red grapefruit
- 1 cup of raspberries
- ½ cup of nectarines, diced
- ½ cup of peaches, diced

- 1 teaspoon to 1 tablespoon of agave syrup (optional)

Procedure:

1. Peel the grapefruit and remove the pith using a sharp knife. Then, slice the fruit in half.

2. Place the grapefruit along with the other ingredients (except the leaves) in a mixing bowl. Add agave and toss.

3. Scoop the mix into the romaine leaves.

3. Killer Kasha Porridge

Kasha is a traditional savory dish popular in numerous countries in Eastern Europe and is usually made from buckwheat. This recipe lets you enjoy this dish in its raw form.

Ingredients:

- 2 cups of buckwheat grouts, soaked and sprouted
- 1 cup of apple, chopped
- 2 teaspoons of orange zest
- 1 tablespoon cinnamon
- ½ teaspoon of sea salt

Procedure:

1. Put all the ingredients in a blender or food processor. Blend until it reaches a porridge-like consistency.

2. Scoop into a bowl and serve.

4. Cinnamon Apple Granola

This enjoyable bowl of crunchy granola is another breakfast favorite. You can change it up and use other fruits such as berries, strawberries or bananas.

Ingredients:

- 2 cups of buckwheat
- 2 apples, cored
- 15 dates, pitted
- ¾ cup of almonds
- ½ cup of cashews
- ¾ cup of Brazil nuts
- 1 ½ cups of sunflower seeds
- ½ cup of pumpkin seeds
- ¾ cup of coconut flakes
- 1 tablespoon of ground cinnamon
- 2 tablespoons of hemp protein powder
- 1 tablespoon of maca powder
- 1 teaspoon of vanilla powder
- ½ teaspoon of salt

Procedure:

1. In a bowl, soak almonds, sunflower seeds, pumpkins and buckwheat overnight. Rinse well before use.

2. In a separate bowl, soak Brazil nuts overnight. Rinse well before use.

3. In another bowl, soak cashews overnight. Rinse well before use.

4. In a food processor, process the Brazil nuts until it achieves a medium fine consistency. Add to the bowl of other seeds and nuts along with the cashews.

5. Add the coconut flakes to the bowl.

6. Process the apples, dates, cinnamon, hemp protein powder, salt, vanilla and maca in the food processor until it gets smooth and saucy. Add to the bowl nuts and seeds. Stir thoroughly by hand.

7. Place layers of the mix on ParaFlexx sheets. Place in a dehydrator at 108°F overnight. If you do not have a dehydrator, use an oven and let it bake until the cashews and almonds are crunchy.

5. Creamy Coconut Yogurt

Yogurt is considered a healing food due to the probiotics it contains which helps colonize the digestive tract. The coconut gives this recipe a creamy backdrop for your fruit or garnish of your choice. Coconuts are also rich in healthy fats, helping you stay full during the day.

Ingredients:

- 2 cups of young Thai coconut meat, shredded
- 1 cup of coconut water
- 1 teaspoon of probiotic powder

Procedure:

1. Place the coconut water and coconut meat in a blender. Blend until creamy.

2. Transfer the mix into a container. Add the probiotic powder and stir.

3. Using a piece of cheesecloth or a towel, cover the container and leave for 4-8 hours to sit at room temperature.

4. Serve in a glass or bowl. Store leftovers in the refrigerator.

Note:

You may choose to add other fruits such as bananas or strawberries to give the yogurt more flavors.

Salads

Being a raw foodist, you probably had someone ask you if salads are all you eat. This is part true; salads are an integral part of the raw food diet and are highly nutritious. But contrary to popular belief, salads are not mundane and flavorless. In fact, here are some delectable salad recipes that you may use.

1. Spiked Citrus Curried Quinoa Salad

Sprouted quinoa is a staple in the raw food diet because it is an amazing source of complete protein. This means it has all the amino acids that the body needs. The addition of the spinach, which provides iron, and the orange juice, which is packed in vitamin C that helps the iron be more absorbable, makes this recipe a very healthy meal.

Ingredients:

- 3 cups of sprouted quinoa
- 4 cups of baby spinach
- 2 scallions, chopped
- ½ cup of orange juice
- 2 tablespoons of olive oil
- 1 teaspoon of curry powder
- ½ teaspoon of coriander powder
- ¾ cup of slivered almonds or pine nuts
- ¾ cup of golden raisins
- ¼ cup of red onion, diced

Procedure:

1. In a large bowl, place the quinoa, onion, raisins and almonds or pine nuts. Toss.

2. In another smaller bowl, whisk the olive oil, orange juice, coriander powder and curry powder together. This will become the dressing of the salad.

3. Drizzle the dressing over the larger bowl of quinoa mixture. Toss completely.

4. Serve the mixture over baby spinach and garnish with scallions.

Notes:

Allow the salad to marinate in the dressing for one hour for better taste.

You may use other dried fruits instead of raisins.

If you want a spicier salad, add sliced jalapeños to the mix.

For a tangier flavor, add tangerine chunks.

2. Lettuce Lover's Salad

If you enjoy greens, then you will love this recipe. This particular recipe emphasizes on lettuce but you can easily change up the recipe and use a different vegetable of your liking such as kale, collards, butter leaf, cabbage, red oak and so much more. After all, variety is the spice of life.

Ingredients:

- 2 cups of romaine lettuce, chopped
- 1 cup of Bibb lettuce, chopped
- ½ cup of red-leaf lettuce, torn
- 1/3 cup of celery, sliced
- ¼ cup of carrots, sliced
- 1 cup of arugula, torn
- 1 cup of endive, torn
- 2 tablespoons of olive oil
- 4 teaspoons of coconut vinegar
- ¼ teaspoon of sea salt
- ¼ teaspoon of agave syrup
- 1/8 teaspoon of onion powder
- 1/8 teaspoon of garlic powder
- 1/8 teaspoon of paprika
- ¼ cup of grape tomatoes, sliced

Procedure:

1. Combine the romaine, Bibb and celery lettuce in a bowl. Add the celery, carrots, arugula and endive. Toss to mix.

2. In a separate bowl, whisk the coconut vinegar, olive oil, agave and all the spices to produce the dressing.

3. Drizzle the dressing over the bowl of salad. Toss thoroughly.

4. Garnish with the grape tomatoes and serve.

3. Sprouted Quinoa, Olive and Tomato Salad

This salad goes well on its own or served with the zucchini hummus on the side.

Ingredients:

- 1 cup of quinoa
- ¼ cup of celery, chopped
- ¼ cup of sun dried tomatoes
- 3/8 cup of sun-dried black olives, pitted
- 2 tablespoons of lime juice
- ¼ teaspoon of salt

Procedure:

1. Soak quinoa for 4 hours. Rinse well before use.

2. Soak the sun-dried tomatoes for 2 hours in water until soft.

3. Dice the tomatoes.

4. Toss all the ingredients in a bowl until thoroughly mixed.

4. Sunset Salad

This colorful salad has a bit of sweetness and a bit of spice and can be enjoyed as an afternoon snack to refuel you. It can also be served with a side of guacamole.

Ingredients:

- 2 cups of romaine lettuce, chopped
- 2 cups of pineapple, cubed
- 1 cup of red-leaf lettuce
- 1 small jalapeño, seeded and minced
- ½ red bell pepper, julienned
- ½ cup of fresh pineapple juice
- 2 tablespoons of apple cider vinegar
- 1 tablespoon of fresh chives, diced
- ¼ teaspoon of sweet paprika
- 1/8 teaspoon of ground black pepper
- 1/8 teaspoon of sea salt

Procedure:

1. In a bowl, place the lettuces, bell pepper and pineapple cubes. Toss to mix.

2. In another smaller bowl, combine the pineapple juice and jalapeño pepper. Add the sea salt, black pepper, paprika and apple cider vinegar to make dressing.

3. Toss the salad with the dressing. Chill the finished product before serving.

4. Garnish with fresh chives and serve.

5. Basic Coleslaw Mix

This is a hydrating coleslaw which you can eat on its own or mix with other dishes. You may also add your own touch to it and add other seasonal vegetables in the recipe.

Ingredients:

- 2 carrots, rinsed and trimmed
- 2 cups of green cabbage, roughly chopped
- 1 ¼ cups of red cabbage, roughly chopped

Procedure:

1. Shred the carrots and both cabbages in a food processor subsequently.

2. Toss all the ingredients in a bowl. Combine well.

Main Courses

The main course is an extremely important part of your daily meal plan. Going on a raw food diet does not necessarily mean that your food choices will be boring and repetitive. In fact, here are some healthy raw food main course recipes that you may easily prepare.

1. Veggie Burger Patties

These patties are not only healthy but are also perfect for people with several food allergies.

Ingredients:

- 3 tablespoons of flax seeds
- 3 to 4 stalks of celery stalks
- 2 carrots, chopped
- ½ cup of onions, chopped
- ½ red bell pepper, chopped
- 1 ½ cups of walnuts
- 3/8 cup of sunflower seeds
- 2 tablespoons of hemp seeds
- 1 tablespoon of protein powder
- 2/3 cup of tomatoes, chopped
- ¾ teaspoon of salt

Procedure:

1. Soak the sunflower seeds and walnuts in water overnight or for at least six hours. Rinse well before use.

2. Using a coffee grinder or blender, grind the flax seeds until powder-like.

3. In a food processor, process the tomatoes, carrots, bell peppers, celery, onions, hemp protein and salt into a puree. Place in a bowl.

4. Process the sunflower seeds and walnuts with along with just the right amount of puree to form a paste. Add this to the rest of the puree in the bowl.

5. Add ground flax seeds and hemp seeds. Mix completely by hand.

6. Form the mixture into patties and place on mesh sheets.

7. Let the patties dry using a dehydrator for at least 18 to 24 hours.

2. Petite Beetloaf

This may serve as a main course for two people and the alternative to the usual meat loaf but with healthier, non-meat ingredients. Despite the lack of meat, it contains a hefty dose of protein due to the walnuts and sprouts.

Ingredients:

- ½ cup of cabbage or mung sprouts
- ¼ cup of alfalfa sprouts
- ¼ cup of beets, shredded
- ½ cup of walnuts, soaked for 2 to 4 hours
- 2 tablespoons of celery hearts, chopped
- 2 tablespoons of white or red onion, chopped
- 2 teaspoons of nama shoyu
- Water

Procedure:

1. Using a food processor, grind the walnuts and sprouts along with the nama shoyu.

2. Add the celery, onion and beets to the food processor and process with a bit of water until all the ingredients stick together.

3. Place this mixture in a sheet and shape into a loaf. Dehydrate at 145°F for at least 12 hours.

3. Spiraled Spaghetti Marinara

The marinara is said to be the dish that truly tests the skills of a chef. This version of the famous pasta is perfect for individuals taking on the raw food diet who are lovers of Italian food. In place of the usual flour, zucchini is used to make the noodles.

Ingredients:

- 3 zucchinis
- ½ teaspoon of salt
- ½ cup of soaked sundried tomatoes, soaked water set aside
- 1 cup of tomatoes, chopped
- ½ cup of red bell pepper, chopped
- 1 clove of garlic, minced
- 2 tablespoons of raisins, dates, chopped apples or currants
- 1 tablespoon of olive oil
- 1 ½ teaspoon of any Italian seasoning
- ¼ teaspoon of cayenne pepper powder

Procedure:

1. If you have a spiralizer, use this to turn the zucchinis into long noodles. Otherwise, you may use a vegetable peeler. Stop until you reach the seeds and get rid of the center.

2. Place the zucchini noodles in a bowl and sprinkle the sea salt on top of it. Stir well. Set bowl aside.

3. Using a food processor or blender, process the sundried tomatoes and the water used for soaking together with all the other ingredients except the noodles. Blend until smooth.

4. Gently squeeze the zucchini noodles to completely get rid of any remaining liquid. Mix with the sauce and toss until thoroughly covered. Serve.

4. Tahini Pad Thai

Pad Thai is among the most recognizable Thai dishes available and is starting to become a favorite all over the world. This national dish from Thailand dates back years ago. The raw version of the Pad Thai replaces the peanuts with sesame tahini, removes the fish sauce, egg and leaves out the noodles for a fresher, lighter and healthier meal.

Ingredients:

- 3 zucchinis, medium
- 2 carrots, large
- ¼ cup of sundried tomatoes, soaked in water
- ½ cup of soak water
- 1 tablespoon of tahini
- 2 tablespoons of nama shoyu
- 2 tablespoons of lime juice
- 1 tablespoon of agave syrup
- ½ cup of snow peas
- ½ cup of mung bean sprouts
- ¼ cup of scallions, finely sliced
- 1 clove of garlic, minced
- ½ tablespoon of ginger
- 2 to 4 tablespoons of cilantro, minced
- Lime wedges

Procedure:

1. In a blender, place together the tahini, nama shoyu, sundried tomatoes, ginger, lime juice, agave syrup and garlic and blend until smooth. While blending, slowly pour in the soak water until the mixture turns thick. This will become your pad thai sauce.

2. Turn the carrots and zucchini into noodles using a spiralizer, mandolin or a peeler. You may choose to grate or julienne them alternatively.

3. On a plate, place your noodles, scallions, snow peas and mung bean sprouts. Add the sauce and garnish with the cilantro and lime wedges.

5. Juicy Hues Stir-Dry

This is a vibrant meal, both for the eyes and the mouth, due to the bright colors of the ingredients and their various strong flavors. This main course has the right amount of saltiness, spice and sweetness that you will surely love.

Ingredients:

- 2 cloves of garlic
- 1 red bell pepper, chopped
- 1 orange or yellow bell pepper, chopped
- 1 mango, cubed
- 1 bunch of broccoli, chopped
- 3 scallions, chopped
- 3 tablespoons of nama shoyu
- 2 tablespoons of orange juice
- 1 tablespoon of lime juice
- 1 tablespoon of olive oil
- 1 tablespoon of hot sauce

Procedure:

1. Whisk together the garlic, nama shoyu, lime juice, orange juice, olive oil and hot sauce in a small bowl. Set aside.

2. In a bigger bowl for mixing, toss the mango, bell peppers and broccoli together. Pour the prepared dressing onto the bowl and thoroughly mix until well-coated.

3. Cover the bowl and let it marinate overnight in the refrigerator or for at least 2 hours at room temperature.

4. After letting it marinate, place the bowl to a dehydrator at 110°F for another 2 hours.

5. Garnish using the scallions and serve.

Conclusion

Thank you again for purchasing this book!

I hope this book was able to help you to get a better idea of the raw food diet and provide you with a vast selection of recipes to assure variety in your diet plan.

Change can be overwhelming at times, especially when you are just about to start out. However, if you do not make the changes that are necessary to make your life better, then you will only continue to hold yourself back. If you want to make improvements to your health and whole well-being, the raw food diet may just be the solution you need.

With the raw food diet, you need not rush into anything. You may take things slow and tinker with your routines until you find the right setup for you. While it may be challenging, the rewards that you will reap will all be worth the sacrifice. Let this book be your starting point in progressing towards a raw and healthy lifestyle.

In addition, please remember to check out our Facebook page in order to find other resources and upcoming promotions:

https://www.facebook.com/joypublishing

With sincere thanks,

Emma Rose

Preview of 'Clean Eating Guide'
Lose Weight Quickly, Achieve Optimal Health and Feel Energized with Clean Eating for Busy Families and Clean Eating Recipes

Chapter 1
What is Clean Eating?

You have probably come across the term 'clean eating' but you are still not familiar about its exact meaning. This is being used by people who work in the health and fitness industry such as personal trainers ad dietitians. People who are health conscious and workout fanatic also often use this word. Does it have something to do with cleaning the food before eating or cooking? Or maybe it has something to do with the kind of food that you eat.

The loose definition of clean eating is eating food in its most natural state. These days, people are starting to pay more attention to the kinds of food that they eat and how these foods are made. They take note of the food's ingredients and make sure that the food product only contains all natural ingredients.

The term clean eating first came out in the 1990s. Today, it is still being used by health conscious individuals from different backgrounds and culture to refer to the kind of all natural diet that they have. The definition of clean eating can vary from person to person. Some define clean eating as eating mostly fruits and vegetables while others define it as not eating anything artificial. You will find out more about these things as you read this book.

What Clean Eating is not?

If you think clean eating is another diet program, like the South Beach diet or Paleo diet, you are wrong because clean eating is a way of life. It also does not follow any strict rules about what food group to eat and not to eat, how many calories you should consume in a meal, and so on. This is the most basic way of healthy eating that promotes weight loss and boost energy. Everybody can do this, even those who are not trying to lose weight.

Clean eating will not make you feel deprived or frustrated because it is so easy to follow. You do not even need to have a really strong determination because it is all a matter of choosing natural over artificial.

Is there such a thing as 'dirty' eating?

You are probably wondering if there is such a thing as 'dirty' eating or the opposite of clean eating. Clean eating does not literally mean eating foods that have less dirt. It means that you are choosing the best and healthiest food choices from different food groups in their most natural state. 'Dirty' eating is not the opposite of clean eating because there is no such thing as eating dirty. The opposite of clean eating is choosing the wrong food to eat and eating junk foods and processed foods that leave toxins in your body.

Clean eating also looks at the source of food. It should not come from large commercial manufacturers that use machines to process food. The foods that clean eaters usually use come from small farms that do not use chemicals and undergo processes. This is why clean eating is often associated with organic eating.

Check out the rest of this book on Amazon or go to: http://www.amazon.com/dp/B00L5FN8RQ/

Check Out My Other Books

Below you'll find some of my other books also available on Amazon and Kindle. Search for these titles on the Amazon website to find them.

Paleo Free Diet Guide for Beginners: Over 50 Paleo Free Recipes for Optimal Health & Fast Weight Loss

Paleo Desserts: Satisfy Your Sweet Tooth With Over 100 Quick & Easy Paleo Dessert Recipes & Paleo Baking Recipes

Raw Food Diet Guide: Lose Weight Quickly, Achieve Optimal Health & Feel Energized with the Raw Food Diet & Raw Food Recipes

Clean Eating Guide: Lose Weight Quickly, Achieve Optimal Health & Feel Energized with Clean Eating For Busy Families & Clean Eating Recipes

Alkaline Diet Guide: Lose Weight Quickly, Achieve Optimal Health & Feel Energized with the Alkaline Diet & Alkaline Recipes

Coconut Flour Recipes for Optimal Health & Quick Weight Loss: Gluten Free Recipes for Celiac Disease, Gluten Sensitivities & Paleo Free Diets

Almond Flour Recipes for Optimal Health & Quick Weight Loss: Gluten Free Recipes for Celiac Disease, Gluten Sensitivities & Paleo Free Diets

Wheat Free Diet for Beginners: Lose Weight Quickly, Achieve Optimal Health & Feel Energized with Gluten Free Recipes for Celiac Disease, Gluten Sensitivities & Paleo Free Diets

Detox Diet Guide: Lose Weight Quickly, Achieve Optimal Health & Feel Energized Through the 10 Day Detox

Sugar Detox Guide for Beginners: Lose Weight Quickly, Achieve Optimal Health, Feel Energized & Eliminate Sugar Cravings Naturally

Ketogenic Diet Guide for Beginners: How to Achieve Rapid Weight Loss, Optimal Health & Unstoppable Energy with Ketogenic Diet Recipes

Anti Inflammatory Diet for Beginners: Lose Weight Fast, Optimize Health, Slow Aging, Fight Inflammation, Conquer Pain & Increase Energy with the Anti Inflammation Diet Recipes

One Last Thing...

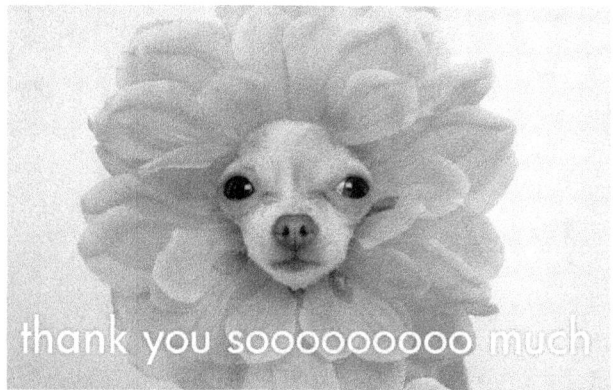

If you believe that this book is worth sharing, would you please take the time to let others know how it affected your life? If it turns out to make a difference in the lives of others, they will be forever grateful to you, as will I.